Essential Fatty Acids

The "Good" Fats

by Deborah Lee

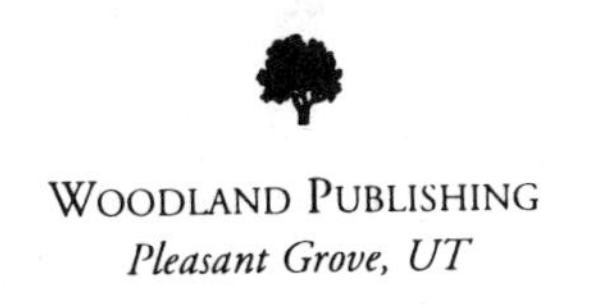

WOODLAND PUBLISHING
Pleasant Grove, UT

Woodland Publishing, Inc.
P.O. Box 160
Pleasant Grove, UT
84062

The information in this book is for educational purposes only and is not recommended as a means of diagnosing or treating an illness. All matters concerning physical and mental health should be supervised by a health practitioner knowledgeable in treating that particular condition. Neither the publisher nor author directly or indirectly dispense medical advice, nor do they prescribe any remedies or assume any responsibility for those who choose to treat themselves.

Contents

Essential Fatty Acids

The "Good" Fats

All About Fats

Some people shy away from anything that has the word "fatty" associated with it. They instantly think it will cause them to gain unnecessary weight. However, there are "good fats" and "bad fats," and the beneficial ones can actually help decrease the desire to eat the harmful ones. Fats are important for health. Also known as lipids, they help balance the body's chemistry and provide padding as protection for vital organs. Fats provide a source of energy for body processes, and they help with the transportation and absorption of fat-soluble vitamins such as A, D, E, and K. They are also a source of the vital nutrients known as essential fatty acids. Categories of fats include the following:

Saturated Fats: All fats are composed of carbon, hydrogen, and oxygen molecules. The carbon atoms of fatty acids hold together in a chain-like fashion. These carbon atoms can attach hydrogen to them. When each place that can hold a hydrogen atom is filled and there is not room for even one more, they are described as saturated. The longer the chain, the harder the fat will be and thus, the higher its melting point. These types of long-chain fatty acids are found in "hard fats," such as those in red meat, butter, cheese, sour cream and palm kernel and coconut oils. When a person's diet is high in saturated fats, these fats tend to clump together in the body and form deposits, along with protein and cholesterol. They then lodge in the cells, organs and blood vessels. This can lead to many health problems, including obesity, heart disease, and breast and colon cancers.

Unsaturated Fats: Unsaturated fats are called such because there are at least two adjacent carbon atoms on a chain which are not attached to hydrogen atoms. When at least two pairs of carbon atoms are empty it is known as a monounsaturated fatty acid. When two or more sets are empty, then it is referred to as a polyunsaturated fatty acid. A good rule of thumb is that the more saturated the fat, the more easily it will stay hard at room temperature.

Essential Fatty Acids: Essential fatty acids (EFAs) are vital nutritional components that our bodies need for many functions. They are found in the seeds of plants and in the oils of cold-water fish. Essential fatty acids—sometimes referred to as vitamin F— cannot be made by the body; they must be supplied in the diet. However, at this time, the government has not officially established a Recommended Daily Intake (RDI). Many factors, including stress, allergies, disease, and a diet high in fried foods, can increase the body's nutritional need for essential fatty acids.

Benefits and Functions of Essential Fatty Acids

The body takes combinations of different triglycerides and makes fats from them to help in various processes. The basic building blocks of any fats are the fatty acids. Fatty acids are either essential or nonessential. A fatty acid is considered essential if 1) the body is unable to synthesize it and 2) the only way it can be obtained is through the diet. In addition, it is considered essential if a deficiency will cause a disease. As far back as 1930 researchers discovered that if an animal did not get essential fatty acids in the diet, it could cause symptoms such as poor reproduction, lowered immunity, rough, dry skin, and slow growth, among others.

There are basically three essential fatty acids. They are linoleic acid, linolenic acid, and arachidonic acid. Linoleic acid is the most vital. Linolenic and arachidonic acids can be converted from linoleic acid, but linoleic acid must be obtained from the diet. Most people are unaware of the many vital functions of essential fatty acids. The list includes:

- Lowering triglyceride levels.
- Helping to eradicate plaque from the walls of arteries.
- Lowering blood pressure.
- Altering the production of leukotrienes which aggravate inflammation in the body. This has shown to be beneficial, especially to those suffering from conditions such as arthritis, lupus, psoriasis and other inflammation-related ailments.
- Constructing body membranes. EFAs work with cholesterol and protein to repair old cell membranes and construct new ones.

- Helping strengthen cell and capillary structures. Fatty acid supplementation in the diet helps replace saturated fats with unsaturated fats. This increases the fluidity of cell membranes, and helps renew their proper function, preventing stiffness and deterioration. The health of the cell membrane depends upon adequate amounts of EFAs.
- Prolonging blood-clotting time, helping wounds to heal. EFAs prevent abnormal blood clotting by inhibiting the production of a substance known as thromboxane, which allows platelets to clot.
- Helping the body manufacture hemoglobin, the compound in the blood that provides oxygen to the cells from the lungs.
- Assisting in the manufacture of cholesterol, while at the same time helping to remove excess cholesterol from the blood. The much maligned body substance known as cholesterol has received a bad rap in the press. Cholesterol, a "waxy alcohol," is actually necessary for many vital bodily functions. It is found in the bile, blood, brain tissue, liver, kidneys, adrenal glands, and myelin sheaths (insulating material) of nerve fibers. It helps the body absorb and transport fatty acids and is necessary for the body to synthesize vitamin D. It is also a building material for hormones produced by the adrenal and reproductive glands. The body will actually manufacture its own cholesterol to ensure a continuous supply of this important fat.

  Cholesterol is synthesized throughout the body. It is manufactured by cells, glands, the small intestine and the liver. Cholesterol is constructed from dietary by-products of proteins, sugars and fats. If the diet contains excessive fats, especially the saturated types, the body will convert them into cholesterol. People who eat high sugar or fat diets may therefore experience elevated cholesterol levels.

- Preventing the growth of bacteria and viruses, which will not thrive in the presence of oxygen, by oxygenating cell membranes. The ability of the highly unsaturated fatty acids to hold oxygen can provide additional benefits such as increasing resistance to disease, endurance, metabolic efficiency, energy conversion, and the balancing of sleep-wake cycles. The entire body is beneficially affected by essential fatty acid nutrition and supplementation. By oxygenation of body tissues, EFAs shorten the exercise recovery time for tired muscles.
- Assisting in the functions of glands and hormones.
- Nourishing skin, hair and nails. EFAs help eliminate eczema, psoriasis, dandruff, and help prevent hair loss. Brittle nails respond to essential fatty acids. EFAs balance the skin's metabolism by controlling the flow of oils and nourish collagen, the supporting structure beneath the skin. Vitamins A and E are fat-soluble and work with essential fatty acids to provide glowing skin and hair.
- Increasing the rate at which the body burns fat.
- Helping the body maintain proper temperature.
- Assisting in the body's production of electrical currents vital for a regular heartbeat.
- Acting as precursors to the production of hormone-like substances called prostaglandins. Gamma linolenic acid especially assists the body with this formation process. Prostaglandins are found in almost all body cells, and act as catalysts for many physiological processes. They help prevent abnormal blood clotting and nerve inflammation. Prostaglandins also help promote blood circulation by dilating the blood vessels and improve immune system function. The most beneficial type of prostaglandin is called PGE-1. PGE-1 balances cholesterol and blood pressure levels, and

stimulates the body's production of T-lymphocytes which strengthen the immune capabilities. Each cell keeps tiny amounts of EFAs and produces prostaglandins from them as they are needed. The name prostaglandins was coined because these substances were originally found in high amounts in the prostate gland. To date, there have been discovered at least thirty-six different prostaglandins with a wide range of roles in the body.

Sources of Essential Fatty Acids

Essential fatty acids are found in both plant and animal sources, although primarily in plants. The EFA family is composed of two main forms, Omega-3 and Omega-6. The following explains exactly what these forms are.

OMEGA-3: The most common forms of Omega-3 are eicosapentaenioic acid (EPA), docosahexaenoic acid (DHA) and alpha-linolenic acid, which comes from plants and helps create EPA and DHA. Omega-3 is usually derived from fish oils. Dr. Roger Illingworth, associate professor of medicine and biochemistry at Oregon Health Sciences University, explains that Omega-3 fatty acids are "long-chained metabolic products from linolenic acid. . . When animals consume and metabolize plants rich in linolenic acid, they produce Omega-3." EPA and DHA are liquid and remain that way, even at room temperature. It is said that they protect fish by providing a body fat that stays fluid even in cold temperatures.

OMEGA-6: The most common form of Omega-6 is is gamma-linolenic acid (GLA). GLA is known to provide the following benefits, among many others:

1. Helps facilitate weight loss in overweight persons (but not in people who do not need to lose any weight).
2. Reduces platelet aggregation (abnormal blood clotting).
3. Helps reduce symptoms of depression and schizophrenia.
4. Alleviates premenstrual syndrome symptoms.
5. May help alcoholics overcome their addiction.

Omega-6 is usually found in plant sources. The oils of cold-water fish such as salmon, bluefish, herring, tuna, mackerel and similar fish are known as Omega-3 fatty acids. The fresh-pressed oils of many raw seeds and nuts contain Omega-6 fatty acids. The most popular sources of Omega-3 and Omega-6 include:

Black Currant Seed Oil: This oil is rich in linoleic acid (44%) and provides almost twice as much gamma-linolenic acid as evening primrose oil. Black currant seed oil also is an excellent source of an Omega-3 precursor known as stearidonic acid.

Borage Oil: This oil comes from *Borago officinalis*, a plant with blue flowers. It is widely recommended in Europe to strengthen the adrenal glands, alleviate symptoms of premenstrual syndrome and relieve inflammation. Besides possibly helping with heart and joint function, it may also assist the growth of nails and hair. Borage oil is also an excellent source of GLA. In *The Complete Medicinal Herbal,* herbalist Penelope Ody asserts that it is "helpful in some cases of menstrual irregularity, for irritable bowel syndrome, or as emergency first aid for hangovers."

Salmon Oil: This oil is high in Omega-3 essential fatty acids. These types of EFAs are known to thin the blood, prevent clotting, regulate cholesterol production and strengthen cell walls, making them less susceptible to viral and bacterial invasion. Salmon oil has a natural ability to help the body relieve inflammation.

In the ground-breaking book *The Omega-3 Breakthrough: The Revolutionary, Medically Proven Fish Oil Diet,* professor Roger Illingworth writes that

> Linolenic acid is a fatty acid with 18 carbons and 3 double bonds. It is manufactured exclusively by plants. When animals consume and metabolize plants rich in linolenic acid, they produce Omega-3. Plankton, a minute form of marine life, is part plant and part animal. Its plant component manufactures linolenic acid. Fish eat the plankton, and the linolenic acid breaks down in their bodies in two types of Omega-3 fatty acids: EPA (eicosapentaenoic acid) and DHA (docosahexaenoic acid) . . . The liquidity of EPA and DHA serves a vital function in fish, who require body fat that remains fluid even in very cold water.

Fish oils, besides containing Omega-3 fatty acids, have shown to benefit those suffering from migraine headaches, arthritis, and high cholesterol levels.

FLAX: Flax is a plant said to date back as far as 5000 B.C. It has been used since approximately 5000 B.C., making it one of the oldest cultivated crops. It is exported from several countries, including Argentina, Canada, India, Russia and the United States. The flowers are usually blue, although they are sometimes white or pink. The mucilaginous seed is, of course, called flaxseed. The oil primarily provides Omega-3/linolenic acid, and provides an average of 57 percent Omega-3, 16 percent Omega-6, and 18 percent of the non-essential Omega-9. Flaxseed oil is said to contain rich amounts of beta carotene (about 4,300 IU per tablespoon) and vitamin E (about 15 IU per tablespoon). In the October 1995 issue of *Let's Live,* the history and uses of flax were highlighted by herbalist Carla Cassata. She writes,

> . . . It's no wonder the Cherokee Indians highly valued the flax plant. They mixed flaxseed oil with either goat or moose milk, honey and cooked pumpkin to nourish pregnant and nursing mothers, providing them with the needed nutrients for creating strong and healthy children. It was also given to people who had skin diseases, arthritis, malnutrition as well as men wishing to increase virility. They believed flax captured energies from the sun that could then be released and used in the body's metabolic process.
>
> This belief has merit. Flaxseed oil, rich in electrons, strongly attracts photons from sunlight. To be effective, EFAs must be combined with protein at the same meal. This flaxseed oil/protein/sunlight combination releases energy and enhances the body's electrical system. Also, this combination, along with vitamin E, can be beneficial for infertile couples and women suffering from premenstrual syndrome . . . Flaxseed oil, having an anti-inflammatory effect on the body, can benefit the 40 million Americans suffering from osteoarthritis and rheumatoid arthritis. To achieve optimum results, however, substances that activate the sympathetic nervous system—like refined sugar, soda, coffee, fluoride—must be eliminated. Stress must also be reduced, because it too, activates the sympathetic nervous system, promoting inflammation.

Evening Primrose: This flower is indigenous to North America, although the oil is particularly popular throughout Europe for therapeutic purposes. It is also known as *night willow* and *evening star.* It is an excellent source of both linolenic and linoleic acids. Both of these nutrients must be obtained from the diet, as the body cannot synthesize them. The seeds contain gamma linolenic acid. This polyunsaturated EFA helps with the production of energy and is a structural component of the brain, bone marrow, muscles and cell membranes. Evening primrose oil has also benefited those with multiple sclerosis, PMS, hyperactivity and obesity. It is estimated that it takes about 5,000 seeds to produce the oil for one 500 mg capsule.

Deficiency Symptoms

Many ailments can be traced to essential fatty acid deficiencies. A lack of linoleic acid in the diet can cause adverse symptoms including:

- Acne
- Changes in personality or behavior
- Gallbladder dysfunction
- Slow healing of wounds
- Cardiovascular problems
- Prostate inflammation
- Thirst due to excessive perspiration
- Arthritis
- Miscarriage
- Poor growth
- Kidney problems
- Muscle tremors
- Skin disorders
- Sterility in males

A lack or low content of linolenic acid in the diet can cause adverse symptoms including:

- Poor growth
- Learning disability
- Tingling in the extremities
- Impaired motor coordination
- Poor vision

Adverse symptoms can disappear when adequate amounts of the deficient fatty acid are given to the person. However, long-term deficiencies of essential fatty acids can cause death. The human body requires forty-five known essential nutrients, and it requires linoleic acid more than any other. Researchers estimate that the body needs at least three to six grams a day, or one to two percent of your daily caloric intake to prevent deficiency symptoms. A much larger amount is helpful to preserve optimum health.

How do you know how much your body needs? The requirements will be different for each person, depending on factors such as stress, diet, and the amount of physical activity you engage in daily. For instance, an obese person who eats a lot of saturated fats will require much more than a thin person who is careful about their dietary intake of saturated fats. A well-balanced diet that includes primary nutrients like vitamins B3, B6, C, zinc and vitamin A will help the body utilize essential fatty acids more efficiently. In his book, *Lipid Nutrition,* Dr. Randy L. Wong states,

> It should be mentioned . . . that the ability of lipids to hold relatively high levels of oxygen has negative implications for the obese. Increased oxygen in fat reserves can result in lipid oxidation and thus free radical formation, which can then increase various tissue pathologies.

This process can be averted by a diet or supplementation regime rich in antioxidant nutrients such as vitamins A, C and E, among others. Several factors can interfere with fatty acid metabolism. They include a diet high in saturated fats and cholesterol, aging, alcohol, high blood sugar, viral infections and aspirin use.

Stay away from fats in which the normal, health-giving properties have been altered to the point where they actually cause damage to the body's cells. Ideally, a health-minded person will not eat deep-fried foods, as these are especially dangerous. However, because we are all human and it is almost impossible to eat a perfect diet nowadays, taking essential fatty acid supplements will help offset the damage done to the body by the "bad fats."

The Danger of Fried Foods

Even natural elements such as light, oxygen and heat can cause the breakdown and rancidity of fats. Recent research has shown that the composition of extremely heated fats, especially those of vegetable origin, may turn into cancer-causing agents by causing free-radical damage to the body. You would think that liquid oils are healthier for you than solid fats. Well, not when it comes to frying. Because solid saturated fats are more stable than liquid unsaturated fats when they are exposed to light, heat and air, they are more desirable than oils for frying. Ideally, we shouldn't really heavily fry food at all, but prepare it like the Chinese do, by stir frying. The Chinese put water into the pan or wok and then the oil, then the vegetables and meat, constantly stirring the mixture around the entire time. This keeps the temperature of the oil lower. It also protects it from oxidation by forming steam which helps keep air from degenerating the oil.

In many commercial restaurants and fast-food establishments, oil is repeatedly reused at high temperatures. It will soon become dark and rancid, exhibiting a strong odor and flavor. Many toxic substances can form when oils are heated to high temperatures. One of these is "trans-fatty acids." These substances are deformed fat molecules which can damage the cells and cause a fatty acid deficiency by inhibiting enzymes that cause fatty acids to be changed into essential molecules. This may, in turn, interfere with prostaglandin production and cause problems with blood pressure and normal platelet action. Ann Louise Gittleman, M.S., underscores the negative impact of commercial oils in her book, *Super Nutrition of Women.*

> Commercially processed oils, hydrogenated margarines, and fried foods—what I call damaged fats—interfere with the transformation of GLA and EPA into prostaglandins. The once-beneficial polyunsaturates have been exposed to processing in the form of excess heat, air, light or hydrogenation that makes them now unusable for the human body. Without the ability to transform into prostaglandins, the EFAs are biologically worthless.

The body cannot use trans-fatty acids so they simply collect around fatty tissues and the body's organs. They also take up space where essential fatty acids normally would be, but do not perform any useful function. It is best to avoid frying food, but when it is necessary, use the Chinese method, or use a small amount of saturated fat (such as butter), and do not heat it to a high temperature.

What About Cooking Oils?

The liquid oils you purchase at the supermarket are exposed to light through the bottles, which causes deterioration. Once you open the bottle, oxygen adds its negative impact. Then, when you heat the oil to a high temperature, it is a detriment to your health. But that is not all. Before it even reaches the supermarket, the oil is already denatured because of the extraction process. If you use oil for cooking, use olive oil.

Mass market refining is concerned with getting the job done as quickly and cheaply as possible. Petroleum (petrochemical) solvents are used to yield the oils from the seeds. Some companies also utilize caustic soda and acid-based clays during the refining and bleaching phases of refining. Following the bleaching stage, harmful substances known as peroxides may form in the oils, as a result of the oxidation and breaking down process.

Believe it or not, the manufacturing process which separates oils from their sources has been employed for more than forty centuries. Modern technology has increased the amount of oil that can be extracted from seed-bearing fruits of flowering plants, and enhanced an oil's shelf life, while saving manufacturing costs. However, this has been at the expense of the aroma, flavor, and nutritional value of the oil.

Sesame seeds are considered to be the first source of extracted oil. More than four thousand years ago, the Assyrians and Chinese would roast the seeds, grind them to a fine powder, and then wait for the oil to separate and rise in the bowl. This took a long time, with very little oil as a result, and this prompted the search for more efficient methods of extracting oil.

Until the 1920s, and even through the early 1940s, oil extraction was conducted on a limited commercial scale, with slow, small, cool-running presses to extract the oil. It was primarily a cottage industry, where flax oil was poured into 100 milliliter bottles and delivered weekly to homes.

In the 1920s, huge oil-producing companies began to emerge. They planted farms where the seeds of specific crops could be processed in huge machines that could press more than 100 tons oil seeds daily by running twenty-four hours a day. Pesticides, synthetic fertilizers and automation increased yields and reduced costs. The negative side was that oils which were previously nutritionally rich were now processed to increase shelf life. Due to this processing, essential fatty acids disappeared from mass-produced oils. There following are signs that reveal the differences between mass-produced and traditional oils.

- You can taste and smell traditional oils. Mass-produced oils are very bland and odorless.
- Traditional oils are produced naturally without pesticides, which can poison the nervous system and interfere with immune function. Mass-produced oils contain pesticide residues.
- Traditional oils are not extracted with solvents. Mass-produced oils may contain residues of these chemicals, many of which may depress central nervous system function and act as lung irritants.
- Traditional oils contain naturally occurring preservatives. Mass-produced oils are kept "fresh" with synthetic antioxidants such as BHT, BHA, citric acid, and methyl silicone. These synthetic antioxidants may interfere with cellular respiration and metabolism. When ingested over a period of years, they may cause degeneration of body systems, leading to disease.
- Traditional oils involve a relative minimum of heat in their production. Lewis Harrison explains, "Mass-produced oils are produced under very high temperatures with loss of many nutritional factors and natural antioxidants. Among those substances removed are lecithin, vitamins A and E, minerals, chlorophyll, and various aromatic and volatile compounds." Free radicals are often found in overly-heated oils. Processing destroys the nutritious components of essential fatty acids and creates what are known as "trans fatty acids." In TFAs, the nourishing structure of fatty acids are changed by heat

and chemicals, the by-product of which are cancer-causing free radicals.

What Are Free Radicals?

Technically, a free radical is an element or molecule with an unpaired electron. If not limited and controlled, they can damage the body's cells and accelerate the processes of disease and aging. Certain enzymes and nutrients, known as antioxidants, will scavenge for free radicals and neutralize them, preventing them from harming the body. They are also known as free radical scavengers. These nutrients include vitamins C and E, beta carotene (provitamin A), grape seed extract, the mineral selenium, and the enzymes glutathione peroxidase and superoxide dismutase (SOD). There are a host of others, including herbs, which are too numerous to mention. Some signs of free radical damage to the body may include premature aging, liver spots, cancer, arthritis and cross-linking which causes wrinkles.

Diet Imbalance

Besides the loss of quality in the production of cooking oils, there are other aspects of our modern world can contribute to imbalanced EFA intake. John Belleme explains in the September/October 1996 issue of *Health Magazine* that

> For most of us, our diets are out of balance when it comes to EFAs. Unlike our ancestors, whose diets were made up of foods containing roughly equal amounts of the two essential fatty acids, Western diets ar short on Omega-3s and too rich in Omega-6s. In fact, the average American diet contains between ten and twenty-five times as much Omega-6 as Omega-3 — far from the ideal

ratio of three to one. How did our diets become so skewed? In large part, it's because we now grow food domestically that is lower in Omega-3s than foods grown in the wild. For example, one researcher found that the eggs of range-fed chickens have a balanced amount of fatty acids, whereas standard United States Department of Agriculture eggs provide twenty times as much Omega-6 as Omega-3. The same disparity is also true of the meat of domesticated pigs, chicken, and cows compared with wild boar, fowl, and deer. Even wild vegetables seem to have more Omega-3s than farm vegetables. In addition, our overconsumption of Omega-6s is partly due to modern food processing, which destroys delicate Omega-3s. At the same time, we are consuming fewer foods that are rich in Omega-3s (such as fish and flaxseeds) and eating more foods that are high in Omega-6s (meat, eggs, and grains). And many of us are eating only vegetable oils that are high in Omega-6s and low in Omega-3s, such as sunflower, corn, sesame, and safflower, which increases our risk of an Omega-3 deficiency.

Many researchers theorize that these radical changes in our diet—most of which have occurred over the last two hundred years—are a major factor in the almost epidemic rates of cardiovascular disease, cancer, and depression these days . . . Although you can remedy a deficiency by taking supplements, don't tip the scale too far in the other direction. Long-term (more than two years) and excessive use (two to four tablespoons a day) of flaxseed or fish oil can cause an Omega-6 deficiency. Once you have eliminated your original Omega-3 deficiency, then concentrate on getting a balance amount of EFAs. Note: When taking EFA supplements, it's important to make sure your diet is rich in vitamins and minerals. Your body needs vitamins A, carotene, B3, B6, C, E, and the minerals magnesium, selenium and zinc to metabolize EFAs . . . Protect your oils. Omega-3 oils usually come in dark bottles but should still always be refrigerated.

Overcoming Disease With EFAs

Studies show that EFAs may be helpful for many chronic, stubborn conditions. The EFAs' ever-growing repertoire of valuable applications includes, among many others, overcoming diseases such as alcoholism, breast cancer and cardiovascular disease, strengthening the immune system, helping eliminate yeast infection, reducing symptoms of premenstrual syndrome, minimizing inflammation of rheumatoid arthritis, and assisting in the proper management of weight.

ALCOHOLISM: Alcohol dependence is a serious condition that can result in decreased life expectancy, suicide, degeneration of the brain and liver, osteoporosis and many other ill effects. The rate at which alcohol is metabolized in the body is different for each person. It has a lot to do with the person's nutritional status, the concentration and activity of certain liver enzymes, and the speed at which the alcohol itself is consumed.

Alcoholics tend not to eat, because the abundant—yet nutrient-poor—calories diminish the appetite. Because of this, alcoholics become extremely malnourished. It is suggested that an overall nutritional program be employed with persons addicted to alcohol. Especially important are vitamins A, C, and B-complex, as well as the minerals zinc, magnesium and selenium. Amino acids (primarily glutamine or glutamic acid), the herb milk thistle, *Lactobacillus acidophilus*, antioxidants, L-carnitine, and the essential fatty acids are also extremely important. Studies show that EFAs, especially those high in gamma-linolenic acid, keep blood lipid levels from going out of control.

Breast Cancer: The body's immune system plays a vital role in protecting us against cancer. Every day, each of us has the potential for getting cancer, but the body's immune system recognizes and annihilates the wayward cells before they have a chance to multiply and do damage. However, when the immune system is overwhelmed or is not functioning properly, the abnormal cells reproduce without anything to stop them. Cancer patients become malnourished and lose weight because the rapidly growing tumors have a voracious appetite for nutrition to keep them going and the person is left with virtually nothing to nutritionally support their health.

There are many natural approaches to preventing breast cancer. Studies show that, among other things, we should have a diet rich in cruciferous vegetables, such as broccoli and cabbage, as well as any food high in fiber. Antioxidants such as grape seed concentrate, vitamins A, C, and E, minerals and essential fatty acids should also be key parts of our daily diet. Research has shown EFAs, especially gamma-linolenic acid (GLA), to have anti-tumor properties.

Cardiovascular Disease: All cells of the body depend upon nutrients transported by the circulatory network. When the blood vessels become clogged with fats and cholesterol, nutrition distribution becomes impeded. When blood flow is stopped in some areas, the heart can die, whether from a sudden heart attack or from gradual weakening over time. Free radicals can damage the linings of the blood vessels, roughening them and making it easier for fat particles to snag and adhere to the blood vessel walls. Some argue that homogenized milk also contributes to blood vessel damage in the same way that free radicals do.

What are some solutions? Exercise is a great way to increase circulation and keep the blood from stagnating. A diet high in fruits, vegetables, natural fiber and low in saturated fats, meats and homogenized dairy products will also help. In addition, antioxidants, hawthorn berry, *Ginkgo biloba*, vitamin E, Co Q-10, L-carnitine, the minerals calcium, magnesium and potassium, and EFAs will also benefit the cardiovascular system.

Studies show that essential fatty acids can help reduce blood pressure and blood fats (lipids), including excessive cholesterol. When fats combine with proteins and carbohydrates, they are called lipoproteins. Lipoproteins are categorized according to the ratio of fat to protein that they contain. High-density lipoproteins (HDL) help the body get rid of excessive cholesterol. Low-density lipoproteins (LDL) do the opposite; that is, they contribute to the accumulation of arterial plaque, or the buildup of cholesterol on arterial walls. If a person has high HDL levels and low LDL levels in their blood, the likelihood of a heart attack is greatly reduced. Omega-3 fatty acids from cold-water fish sources raise the level of HDL in the blood.

Immune System: A healthy immune system, the body's defense fortress against disease, depends upon a holistic approach. A positive mental attitude alone can do much to boost the body's resistance to illness. Conversely, depression and worry can debilitate the body's defenses. A nutritious diet which emphasizes fresh, raw fruits and vegetables, whole grains and herbs can go a long way toward ensuring that the immune system operates at peak capability. The herbs echinacea, uña de gato, pau d' arco, golden seal, garlic; the minerals zinc and selenium; and vitamin C work to help nourish the immune system. It is thought that EFAs enhance the body's immune system activity by stimulating macrophage and lymphocyte responses.

There are specific nutrients known to enhance immunity to disease. Anne Louise Gittleman, M.S., in her book *Super Nutrition for Women,* explains,

> There are 45 essential nutrients that are critical for total body function. These include 20 minerals, 15 vitamins, 8 amino acids (the building blocks of protein), and 2 fatty acids (the building blocks of fat). These nutrients cannot be made from other substances; we must get them in the natural state from foods or, in some cases, dietary supplements. We need a balance of the proper essentials for the regulation of every function in the human body. From the original Omega-3 fatty acid (alpha-linolenic acid), our bodies make eicosapentaenoic acid (EPA) and docosahexaenoic acid (DHA). From the original Omega-6 fatty acid (linoleic), our bodies produce gamma-linoleic acid (GLA). These two series of essential fatty acids are found naturally in cold-water fish rich in Omega-3 and unprocessed vegetable, seed, and botanical oils rich in Omega-6. Both groups must be provided by the diet because the body cannot produce them itself.
>
> Once known as vitamin F, these essential fatty acids (EFAs) must be present in the diet along with vitamin E and the B vitamins to produce sex and adrenal hormones and control cell growth. The benefits credited to polyunsaturates are actually the health benefits provided by the essential fatty acids or EFAs.
>
> For example, the EFAs are a component of the outer membrane of every cell, where they protect against invading viruses, bacteria, and allergens. Flexibility and fluidity of the cell membrane depend on the presence of the EFAs. EFAs increase metabolism and energy production. They help dissolve body fat into body fluids (yes, fat to lose fat!), decreasing blood cholesterol and triglyceride levels. They distribute the fat-soluble vitamins A, D, E, and K throughout the body, insulate the nerves, and help maintain equal body temperature.

> Essential fatty acids are also the building blocks from which prostaglandins are made. These hormone-like substances regulate every organ, tissue, and cell in the human body at a basic cellular level. . . . One type stimulates production of thyroid hormone, assuring the energy we need. Prostaglandins also block your body's production of histamine, the chemical responsible for the itching eyes, stuffy nose, and scratchy throat in an allergic reaction. Decreased levels of prostaglandins may bring on some types of asthma; researchers know that if levels are adequate, muscles in the lungs relax and blood flow increases. Prostaglandins have proven helpful in relieving various premenstrual (PMS) symptoms as well as depression and conditions ranging from arthritis and ulcers to migraines and cancer.

Candida Yeast Infection (candidiasis): Essential fatty acids inhibit the growth of yeast organisms in the body by helping the oxygen flow to cells. Yeast is anaerobic and cannot thrive in the presence of oxygen. Yeast overgrowth can cause a multitude of symptoms that may be diagnosed as some other ailment. They range from allergies and throat infections to joint swelling and memory loss.

Premenstrual Syndrome: PMS is actually a collection of symptoms which occur one to two weeks before menstruation. It generally affects about one-third of women who are younger than forty years of age. It is caused by hormone imbalances; primarily, the body's overproduction of estrogen and a subsequent deficiency in progesterone. Excessive estrogen causes increased levels of important neurotransmitters such as adrenaline, noradrenaline and serotonin. It can also decrease amounts of dopamine and phenylalanine. This imbalance can result in anxiety, irritability, and mental sluggishness. Excessive estrogens can also inhibit the action of B6, prevent the liver from synthesizing serotonin and causing a hypoglycemic (low blood sugar) condition. They also inhibit the body's release of endorphins, substances which have mood-elevating and pain-relieving properties.

Fluid retention in the face, hands and ankles can result from an overproduction of the hormone adosterone. PMS is also caused by an increased production of the hormone prolactin. Research shows that women with PMS usually consume more refined carbohydrates, dairy products and sodium and less iron and other minerals than women who are symptom-free.

Nutrients which are very helpful for PMS include vitamin B complex, beta carotene and vitamin E, minerals (especially magnesium), a mineral supplement, the herb milk thistle (to help the liver process and eliminate excessive estrogen), *Lactobacillus acidophilus* and essential fatty acids. Essential fatty acids (especially GLA) help to balance the body's hormone levels.

RHEUMATOID ARTHRITIS: The etiology, or cause, of rheumatoid arthritis is currently the topic of scientific scrutiny. Possibilities range from inherited predisposition, diet, food allergies and bacteria. The strongest evidence points to intestinal permeability, bacterial antigens and imbalances in intestinal flora. Translated, this means that the walls of the intestinal tract are weak and bacteria and poisons which otherwise would be kept from absorbing through the intestinal walls, pass through, get into the bloodstream and cause autoimmune flare-ups in the body. This is sometimes referred to as the "leaky gut syndrome." Toxins subsequently find a cozy home in the bowel area and further multiply, crowding out the "friendly" bacteria.

Diet has been suspected as one of the culprits in rheumatoid arthritis because in cultures where fruits, vegetables and fiber are the mainstays, rheumatoid arthritis is virtually unknown. Eating a lot of sugar, meat, refined carbohydrates and saturated fat seems to aggravate rheumatoid arthritis.

Allergies to foods such as wheat, dairy products, corn, and foods in the nightshade family (such as green peppers, potatoes, tomatoes, and eggplant) have been linked to symptoms for many with rheumatoid arthritis.

The nutritional approach to rheumatoid arthritis includes taking the herbs uña de gato (cat's claw), devil's claw, licorice root, siberian ginseng; digestive enzymes and betaine HCl; amino acids, selenium, vitamins E and C, bioflavonoids, zinc, manganese, *Lactobacillus acidophilus*, shark cartilage, glucosamine sulfate, and essential fatty acids. Cayenne pepper extract or cream, applied topically to the painful area, has helped many rheumatoid arthritis sufferers with temporary relief of inflammation and pain.

Essential fatty acids (especially gamma-linolenic acid) help to mitigate or decrease internal inflammation. GLA changes quickly to dihomogamma-linolenic acid (DLA) in the body, which is then converted to prostaglandin E1 (PGE 1), a potent anti-inflammatory substance. The effectiveness of essential fatty acids in helping rheumatoid arthritis has been validated through modern science. Scientists at the University of Pennsylvania conducted research on gamma-linolenic acid and rheumatoid arthritis. They gave 1,100 mg of GLA per day from borage seed oil to seven patients. Six out of the seven experienced reduced synovitis (inflammation of the synovial fluid in joints). In a later 24 week trial study, 14 rheumatoid arthritis patients took 1,400 mg daily of GLA from borage seed oil capsules. Thirteen patients were given a placebo. The following results were noted: In the GLA patients, the number of tender joints decreased by 36 percent. The degree of tenderness was reduced by 45 percent and stiffness of joints upon arising diminished by 33 percent. The placebo patients did not get better or worse.

Obesity: Essential fatty acids help dissolve body fat and increase metabolism and energy production. Ann Louise Gittleman, M.S., author of *Beyond Pritikin* says, "EFAs help burn excess calories instead of depositing them as fatty tissue. They also act as solvents to help the body dissolve and remove hard fats. Craving fatty foods can indicate an EFA deficiency." Brown fat is a unique tissue inside the human body that actually helps the body burn fat to create heat and energy, instead of depositing excess calories for storage as fat. Gamma-linolenic acid (found especially in evening primrose oil and borage oil) activates brown fat metabolism. If a person is 10 to 20 percent above his ideal body weight he is considered overweight. Obesity is considered by some health experts to be America's foremost health problem. It is estimated that 25 to 45 percent of adults over thirty are overweight.

The simple answer to maintaining your weight is to expend as many calories as you take in. To lose weight, your caloric intake must be less than the amount that you expend. If your goal is to gain weight, your caloric intake must exceed the energy you utilize. Your body will store as fat any excess, unused calories.

Try to maintain a your weight by eating a healthy diet and exercising regularly. As you age, your metabolism will naturally slow, and you may have to adjust your diet and exercise routine.

Conclusion

The essential fatty acids are truly the welding link in nutritional health. Simple deficiencies can cause symptoms which may be mistaken for major systemic diseases such as diabetes. Essential fatty acids provide many health-giving properties which positively impact human vitality. Their myriad benefits include regulating blood pressure, nourishing the immune system, controlling inflammation in the body and preventing the formation of abnormal blood clots.

References

Fast, Julius; *The Omega-3 Breakthrough Fish Oil Diet;* The Body Press; Tucson, Arizona; 1987

Gittleman, Ann Louise, M.S..; *Super Nutrition for Women*; Bantam Books; New York; 1991,

Ody, Penelope; *The Complete Medicinal Herbal;* Dorling Kindersley; New York, 1993.

Wong, Dr. Randy L.; *Lipid Nutrition: Understanding fats and oils in health and disease;* Inquiry Press; Midland, Michigan; 48640

Harrison, Lewis; *The Complete Fats and Oils Book;* Avery Publishing Group; Garden City, New York; 1990, 1996.

Harrison, Lewis; *Making Fats & Oils Work for You;* Avery Publishing Group; Garden City, New York; 1990.

Bang, H.O.; Dyerberg, J.; *Plasma Lipid and Lipoprotein Pattern in Greenlandic West-Coast Eskimos;* Lancet 1(1971):1143-6.

Prescott, S.M.; "The Effect of Eicosapentaenioic Acid on Leukotriene B Production by Human Neutrophils"; *Journal of Biologic Chemistry;* 259(1984): 7615-21.

Kaunitz, H. and Johnson, R.E.; "Influence of dietary fats on disease and longevity"; (1975) *Proceedings of the Ninth International Congress of Nutrition* (Mexico, 1972). Vol. 1 ed. by A. Chavez, et al. Basel, Switzerland: 369.

"Dietary essential fatty acids, prostaglandin formation and platelet aggregation": *Nutrition Reviews* 34:243.

Corbett, R.; Berthou, F.; Leonard, B.E. and Ménez, J.F. 1992. "The effects of chronic administration of ethanol on synaptosomal fatty acid composition: modulation by oil enriched with gamma-linolenic acid." *Alcoholism* 27:11.

Cantrill, R. C., Ells, G., Chisholm, K. and Horrobin, D.F. 1993. "Concentration -dependent effect of iron on gamma-linolenic acid toxicity in ZR-75-1 human breast tumor cells in culture." *Canc. Lett.* 72:99.

Das, U.N. 1992. Anti-cancer effects of cis-unsaturated fatty acids both in vitro and in vivo. *Lipid-Soluble Antioxidants: Biochemistry and Clinical Applications.* Ong, A.S.H. and Packer, L., Eds. Birkhauser Verlag, Basel, Switzerland, p. 482.

Takeda, S., Horrobin, D., Manku, M., Sim, P.G. and Simmons, V. 1992. Propose lipid peroxidation mechanism for selective destruction of breast cancer cells in culture by gamma-linolenic acid (GLA). In: Oxygen Radicals. Proceedings of the 5th International Congress on Oxygen Radicals: Active Oxygen, Lipid Peroxides and Antioxidants. Kyoto, 17-21 November 1991. Yagi, Kondo, M., Kiki, E. and Yoshikawa, T., Eds. Elsevier Science Publ. B.V., Amsterdam, p. 277.

Takeda, S., Horrobin , D.F. and Manku, M.S. 1992. "The effects of gamma-linolenic acid on human breast cancer cell killing, lipid peroxidation and the production of Schiff-reactive materials". *Med. Sci. Res.* 20:203.

Engler, M.M. 1993. "Comparative study of diets enriched with evening primrose, black currant, borage or fungal oils on blood pressure and pressor responses in spontaneously hypertensive rats." *Prostaglandins Leukotrienes Ess. Fatty Acids* 49:809.

Singer, P., Naumann, E., Hoffman, P., Block, H.U., Taube, C., Heine, H. and Forster, W. 1984. "Attenuation of high blood pressure by primrose oil, linseed oil and sunflowerseed oil in spontaneously hypertensive rats." *Biomed. Biochim. Acta* (8/9):243

Ockerman, P.A., Bachrack, I., Glans, S. and Rassner, S. 1986. "Evening primrose oil as a treatment of the premenstrual syndrome". *Recent Adv. Clin. Nutr.* 2:404.

Leventhal, L.J., Boyce, E.G. and Zurier, R.B. 1993. "Treatment of rheumatoid arthritis with gammalinoleic acid". *Ann. Int. Med.* 119:867.

Tate, G., Mandell, B.F., Laposata, M., Ohliger, D., Baker, D.G., Schumacher, H.R. and Zurier, R.B. 1989. "Suppression of acute and chronic inflammation by dietary gamma linolelinc acid." *J. Rheumatol.* 16:729.

Garcia, C.M., Carter, J. and Chou, A. 1986. "Gamma linolenic acid causes weight loss and lower blood pressure in overweight patients with family history of obesity". *Swed. J. Biol. Med.* 4:8.